bellyache

Also by Brianna Pastor

Good Grief

bellyache

poems for sensitive souls

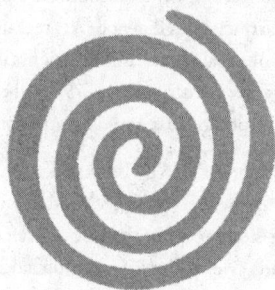

brianna pastor

HarperOne

An Imprint of HarperCollins*Publishers*

HarperCollins books may be purchased for educational, business, or sales promotional use. For information, please email the Special Markets Department at SPsales@harpercollins.com.

harpercollins.com

FIRST EDITION

Illustrations by Natalia Skeba
Designed by Yvonne Chan

Library of Congress Cataloging-in-Publication Data has been applied for.

ISBN 978-0-06-345910-6

Printed in the United States of America

25 26 27 28 29 LBC 5 4 3 2 1

To those who deeply feel and
don't know what to do with it.
You are not alone.

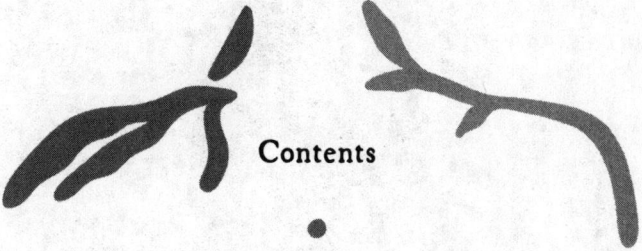

Contents

·

Author's Note
ix

Body
1

Mind
39

Soul
97

Acknowledgments
143

Author's Note

From the moment I could think, I have always had this inner knowing that I wasn't "from" here, or that I didn't "belong" here. And not in the depressing kind of way; I just knew that something about me was different, and I could never put my finger on it. What I did know is that everything weighed on me, heavily. My grandmother would tell me stories of how, when I was a child, I would awaken in the middle of the night, stare off blankly into space, and then burst into uncontrollable crying. She used to say I could feel all the sadness of the world (and in my own world, whether it tried to be hidden from me or not) and didn't know what to do with it. And she was right. I could never tell her why I was crying so much, but I also couldn't stop.

I did research on children who felt they didn't belong here. I came across a concept called "Indigo Children," before I ever knew what an empath was. This concept made the most sense to me, because I was highly sensitive and intuitive and felt like I could feel aspects of a different universe. I was born knowing that this, here on Earth, is not all there is. I could feel it in my bones. I just . . . knew.

My sensitivity has not been accepted by most people—as a child and even now, as an adult. It was weaponized against me for most of my life and made me an easy target for being taken advantage of. After being severely bullied in school and finding it difficult to make friends, I was convinced that my sensitivity was a curse. I thought it was the thing that was irreparably wrong with me, and everyone could see it. And while being highly sensitive can be extremely difficult, it is also the most beautiful thing you can be. As an adult, I know this now.

I've come to realize that being an empath isn't about the trauma I have endured. Your innate ability to connect and feel things beyond what others can see is a gift that can only be expanded through experiencing hardship. Anyone can exercise their empathy muscle, but very few people are born with the natural ability to pick up emotions, energy, physical ailments, other-worldly elements. We connect to the world on a different level than most people and because of this, we also tend to suffer just as deeply. It is no easy feat—to feel so misunderstood in a world we carry the weight of, and we certainly don't get to decide to just "put it down." The gift of feeling so deeply is something that makes us, us. And I believe we are meant to heal as much of the world as we can.

To do this, we must learn how to exist and accept ourselves as sensitive souls. This world has become increasingly harsh, no matter what walk of life you have experienced. We were not meant to see or feel this much pain, but here we are. And although I have not yet figured out how to manage it well, the least I can do is remind you that you're not alone. And that you belong here, and that we need you.

I hope *Bellyache* can remind you that there are other sensitive souls in the world who feel and think the way you do. Feeling this deeply can be such an isolating experience and it isn't the easiest concept to explain to others. The older I've gotten, the more I've come to realize that I don't need to explain my heart to others. Some people will see you and others won't be able to.

I hope this collection is the friend you need sitting beside you when the feelings are just too overwhelming. I hope it can hold you the way that you need, whenever you need it. As you read, please remember: nobody can tell you who you are if you already know. And nobody can take away your capacity to feel. That is the thing deeply embedded within you that more of the world could benefit from.

If you feel it all, I'm right there with you.

Briana Pastor

From my debut collection, *Good Grief*,
the poem that inspired this book:

I don't want to
grow a thick skin

I want my skin
to stay
as thin as it was made
and
everything outside of that

to be softer

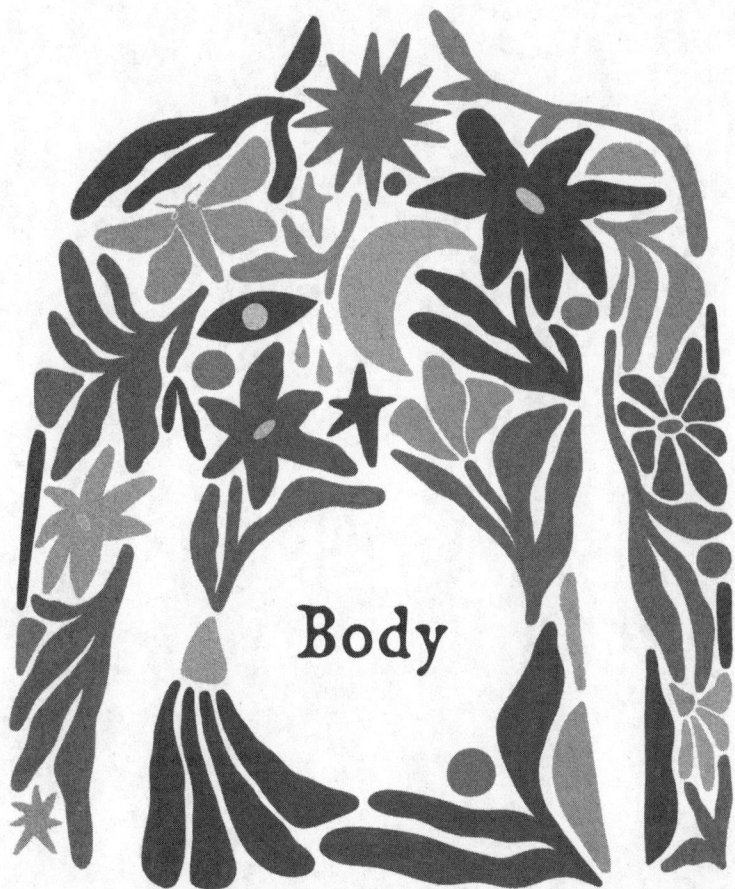

Body

At night I build forts with my shadows.
I pin the corners of the sheet to the ceiling like
fragile anxiety waiting to snap off at any given
moment.
I let the ends droop at my sides, covering just enough
of me;
sadness now contained to the small vicinity I lie in.
I feel weak, my head is still but my world is spinning
and I feel the heart attack happening from across the
country.
In the moments I lie here, I feel the loss of a sister
and a family and a population and a life.
I feel the poverty, the bone-chilling abuse,
I feel the thoughts before the noose.

If I was really having a heart attack, I'd be dead by now.
I feel every single thing I have ever been through
and every single emotion that exists outside of myself,
as this simultaneous breath leaves my mouth
and drifts away into the sheet above my face.
I feel so much pain.

I say that I can't possibly contain this much,
and I surprise myself every time.

It took me thirty years to realize, but,
most of this pain I have carried
was not my own.

There are red freckles forming on my sternum;
I have lost count since they began to spread
and everyone around me is dying.
Somewhere on this hill
I have died, lived several times,
and I'm still not sure if I've done it well.
And no, don't say that time will tell,
because there are humans believing that
queer lives are a sin—there are battles to win.
And I can't climb down this hill until I've
planted my feet deep enough to say: I've tried.
I've made
        a small dent,
              a ripple effect,
changed someone's mind.
Made this world a little more loveable.
Is that a lot to carry? Is that
too big of an ask?
For people to acknowledge the
blip of time we exist in
and ask them to do
anything
to make it a little more worth staying?

(Thump, thump, thump . . .)

Can you feel it? That thing in your chest?
It is quite literally begging you to care for it.

(Please, please, please . . .)

When there is a fire in your stomach,
ask:
Does this hurt? Do I feel alive?
From experience, the first is usually anger,
the latter—your inner power.
Harness the power and
let the anger course through
but never confuse the two;
and certainly never let them walk into
the same room without introducing them.

It might be five o'clock somewhere,
but it's one in the morning here now.
I have always been a night owl;
sleep was never an invitation, but an exhaustion.
Night-time is when my body decides
it will gather all of my things and set out
to relive every memory.
One does not just simply lie down; I must
lie facing the door—just in case.
I must listen for every sound even if
it's just the house settling instead of my anxiety.
But even after the locks are checked six times
and the lighting is a calm sort of dim, my body
is fighting for its reconciliation. Its stillness.
But the shaking inside my body feels
like it has grown its own pulse and
I can't help but wonder
if I'll ever see the day when it gets up and
walks away from me.

There are days you will feel in your bones.
You will wake to find that night carried itself

into the morning without warning, asking you
to hold a little more than you had bargained for.

There will be a lot of days.
Some that will hurt, some that lift the worry—

and on both days, you mustn't let the painful fog
of guarded memories creep up your sternum

and change your face. You mustn't wear the fog
like a tight cape tied at the neck. Instead,

pull it out of your throat and hold it in your palm,
giggling because it was much smaller than it felt.

I have a bellyache
from constantly absorbing
all this pain.

I'd ask you to refrain from telling me,
but your eyes already have.

I never made much sense to anybody.
Always running around yards
finding the carcass of something once alive,
only to give it a proper burial.
The girl who cries at the first sign of trouble,
but always finds herself in it.

I don't know why I choose
to make papier-mâché out of life and
call it an escape—
glue it to the inside of my eyelids
and pray that what I see is my reality.
I don't know much, but

It stings. It stings. It stings.

Maybe one day
the sun will dance off the sky
and land under my eyelids—

The moon will spontaneously
combust
and join my belly in
its fullest shape.

Flowers will give praise
in my direction
for staying intact
in these harsh conditions.

Or something else resembling
what others expect of me.

Let me rummage through my soft fire of a life
without rushing to put it out.

Your body is wise—it knows many things before you do. Before others do, even. It can be difficult to tell the difference between your anxiety and your intuition. Learn to pay attention to the way your body reacts around people, how it feels when someone leaves your life. It may hurt, but does your body blossom? Do you feel a sense of relief?

Listen to this: your heart can hurt, but your body is already preparing you to heal, all in the same breath. There is something deeply rooting for your alignment before you have a chance to figure it out for yourself. And when we ignore it, we eventually learn the hardest way. So, sit in the hurt, but the relief your body simultaneously feels is saying,

"Hey, you are going to be okay."

The only way to make you understand
a sensitive heart is to have you imagine
nerve endings on the outside of your skin.
Open, exposed—and maybe this is why
skin is *soft* and often mistaken for thin.
Because there is nothing above it
that protects the world from getting in.

My hands have always been a
pretty good read of who I am:
shaky, warm and unsure.
Maybe that's why they always say
your heart is the size of your fist.

I think most people see a person who is bright and a little bit bruised, kind of like the way we see a peach ready to be eaten alive. I think they see the color changing as a quirk, something to try out. But when they bite into it, they realize there was a lot more "gone bad" than they had ever thought.

And like all good things that are a little too touched by life, they throw you away without a thought. But just because I am soft and changing doesn't mean I don't deserve to be savored. That's where the juice is.

If ever you find yourself stuck
between your heart and your mind,
sit under the tree.

The wind will remind you that
everything moves.
The ground will remind you that
you are steady.
The sky will remind you that
change is happening with you.
The rain will teach you
to adapt.

And even if there is no body of water near,
you can almost hear it.
That is the sound of
your body coming back to you.

Frantic and afraid,
I have learned that my body
dances one way or another.
Whether it is fleeing panic or
intentional rhythm—
I will never just lie down and surrender.

I hold my pain
in my stomach and
it gives me the guts
to write about it.

Every day I change. Glance
at my tired face and wonder
when I'll resemble something
that looks like bravery—
someone who doesn't wear their
heart on their face
for the world to punch.
A beating of sorts.

I hold grief in the small of my back.
I keep bending over backwards
attempting to release it.
That's probably why you feel
a sudden urge to cry
any time you hug me.
Maybe your hands can hear
the crack in my spine's voice.

I am tightly-wound
in a way that would put
anxiety to shame.

My bones know secrets
that have never been said out loud.
They know what might happen
and what has already happened
and everything that could
possibly go wrong.
And that is why they are always aching,
always one secret away from breaking,
never healing the way they're supposed to.
And maybe you'll believe me when I say:
I'll take your secrets to my grave.
So when all that's left of me is bone,
you are all that remains.

To cry
means that you are feeling
as much as you possibly can
in that moment.
And that is exactly what I mean
when I say that
you are alive.

I feel all my emotions
to my very core. Some,
I suppress. Some, I allow.
Either way, each one
lives within me.
I don't get to re-home them,
but I do get to know them well.
And what a miraculous thing—
to know many things so deeply
that you learn how to nurture them.
But sometimes I hide in my room
and keep the door locked.
This, too, is part of the process.
You can exist in the same house,
but you can't let them control your space.
So, lock your door sometimes.
But always come back out.

Your legs may be an earthquake.
Heart like a twister,
your tongue, at times, becomes the Sahara.
Maybe thoughts turn into a cyclone.
You are not much different than nature.
You are also the morning sun
on the first day of spring,
the steam that rolls off the fresh coffee.
Your genuine nature oozes out
and everyone around you can breathe easier for it.
Aurora Borealis the way you effortlessly
change like you were born to do it.
You must see the good of the world
and the good in you,
everything else is just
the nature of things. So remember,
you are not bad, no.
You are a wonderful collection
of what it means to be alive
at the same time as everything else.

I used to joke that you could tell
how much I'd been through from
how thin I was growing up.
I was the definition of frail,
as thin as the amount of love
I'd experienced.
And once I finally felt real love,
I knew what it was to be full.
Filled with laughter, and ease—
safe enough to devour the things
I had once feared would kill me.

I can't remember a good portion of my life. But I can tell you every instance I lay awake, begging from my stomach that someone would rescue me. My grandmother used to tell me that even when I was a toddler, I would wake in the middle of the night and just start crying. The inconsolable kind. I would stare into space for minutes at a time and burst into tears. I could hear how piercing the silence was. I knew what it meant. I knew that the quiet was because there was no love there. And I didn't know how to fix it.

I find myself wanting to
stretch this skin
over your body
and live your pain for you.

Every time you held my hand,
you'd turn your head the other way.
You'd roll your eyes to the back of your head
and take a deep sigh disguised as a breath.
I want you to know,
I could feel that.

I have met every kind of tear.
The silent, the slow, the ones that
come for no reason at all. The loud,
the painful, the ones that slip down
the side of your face into your ears.
The friend, the ones that never leave
the pillowcase. The ones you hide.
And when I met each of them, I
already knew of their taste. They say
salt in the wound hurts, and they
aren't wrong. But what's a brief
sting when you have seen relief
first-hand? To know that the wound
is a type of tear in and of itself, one that
will seal but not without blistering first.
An other-worldly reminder that an
emotion does come to life,
right before these very eyes.

Your spark will go out again.
This, I know.
This comes with the territory
of being so deeply in tune
with everything around you.
With having so much empathy
that goes unguarded.
But the good news? When it
comes back on, when the light
kneels behind your eyes again,
you'll remember both versions
of you. And you'll get to decide
which one needs the shield.

You must abandon every single judgment that exists in your mind. Most of what holds us back is the fear of what those around us will think. If we continue to allow this to guide our personal decisions, we will continue to find ourselves stuck. Let us dismantle the need to satisfy others. We are living for what we can be and feel and do in this life. We must do as we feel in our stomachs. There is life ahead of us, waiting to be devoured and inhaled and touched. There is more out there. And by then, we will laugh at the silly judgments, proud they did not determine our trajectory. Singing at the taste of what it feels like to mend.

I can't eat because
I know the world is hurting.
My stomach hurts in anticipation
of something I suspect may happen
tomorrow.
And my chest; oh, my chest—
She knew you would betray me
long before I did.
My body warned me and I did not listen.
My body healed me and I did not appreciate.
Everything beautiful and free
flew at the speed of light, right past me.
It's hard to see the roses
with the thorn already in your side.

Leave me in silence—
to find the answers I have been
begging all my life for. To reach
deep within my aching body
and teach myself how to
mend. How to breathe again.
How to wring out the pain
I've absorbed and return
back to myself in full.

Some days,
when the sun comes out
and the air is warm,
your heart will still
feel buried under
what winter left behind.

I feel what you feel
in my bones—

and I'm not quite sure
where it all goes.

Sometimes, when the energy
in the room becomes so dense,
I can feel my throat closing.
I feel my heartbeat in my feet
and suddenly I forget how to walk.
Sometimes, stepping into a crowded room
means stepping into a room filled with
everyone's childhood traumas.
You see a body, I feel a small child
crying, begging, pleading—
and you wonder why I always
need to leave.
I can't muster up the courage
to brave the small talk
when my body is screaming,
"You deserved so much better,
I'm so sorry."

My heart is not a neatly wrapped
Christmas gift nor a well-hosted
house-warming party. It is a scream,
a warm bath, legs flailing in the air
as it runs. A whimper, a three-hour-long
meltdown, the anglerfish at the
very bottom of the ocean. My heart
is battle and safety and something that
doesn't make sense in this world.
It is a birthday party that went
extremely wrong.
So, grab some confetti and
a piece of cake and come
cry on the floor with me.

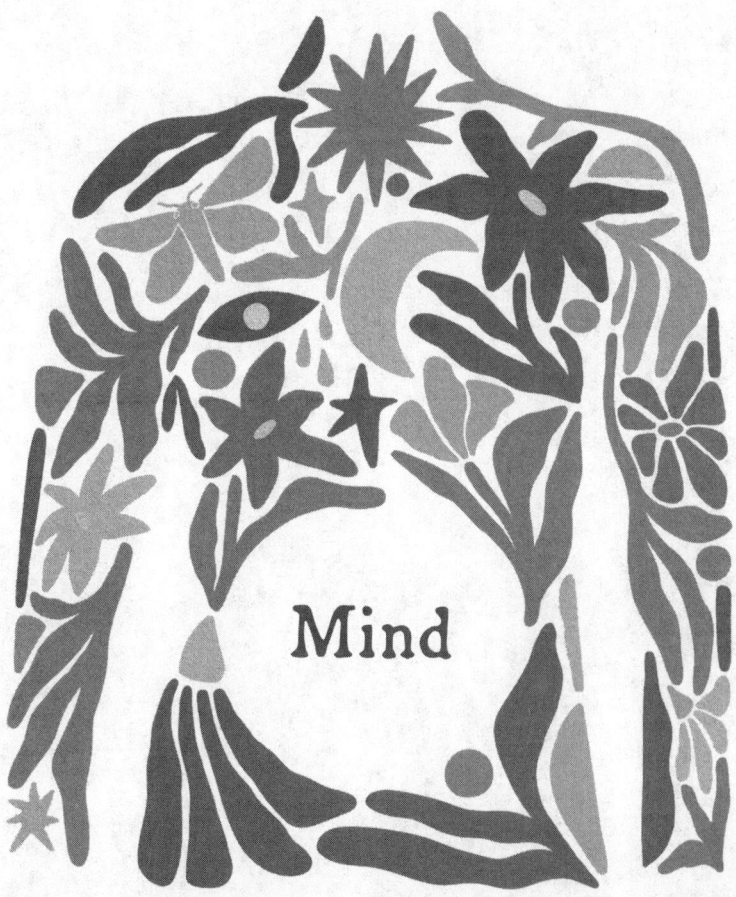

Mind

The amount of heartache I've saved myself from
is equivalent to the amount I've endured, you know.
I've untangled decades of webs, tried to reverse the
generational trauma I was so graciously gifted.
The alcoholic gene must have slipped through the cracks
when everything was transferred over.

I've said so often: it ends here.
But it was never as easy as they made it seem.
How do you heal for *the rest of your life?*
Part of me tried, *really tried,*
and the other part doesn't want to let it go.
Because I fear that someone, someday,
at the end of it all
will ask me: *how deeply did you love?*
And I'll have nothing to show for it.

Maybe this life of mine won't be loud and praised.
Maybe it will be wilted and dried out for decoration,
whiffs of flowers every time I pass through the room.
It will be hot coffees and check-ins and friends
passing through like a train station and
teaching someone how to care for themselves
because their family never did.
It will be coming to fully understand how to love others
because of the love I found myself.
Maybe it will be learning from that love.
It will be a canopy of safety and comfort that I
couldn't otherwise find in the world, filled with
books written by brilliant minds and maybe
I know some of them.
It will be subtle, with a lack of chaos,
And maybe that is loud enough for me.

We only desperately try to save in others
what we fear to lose within ourselves.

We only desperately try to give to others
what we want to see within ourselves.

At the end of my road,
a color-blind man paints
his house yellow,
the only color he is able to see.
It became the brightest yellow
I have ever personally seen,
mostly because you can
feel him shine through it.

Could life still
be as sweet
if it did not sometimes
Sting?

If I let go, and I mean *really* let go
of my fear,
I am afraid it will end up
in somebody else's head.

Come out, come out,
wherever you are.
You were taught to hide,
little one—
Someone taught you that hiding
was your best chance at surviving
but they were wrong.
They were so wrong.
How are we ever supposed
to love that extraordinary heart
if you keep it tucked away
behind a curtain
so that the light
can never shine on it?

It's safe to come out,
but just in case you're scared:
I'll never stop looking.

Morning peaks through the window
like a birth, asking me to prepare and adjust
and give it a beautiful name.
Mid-day approaches and I find myself
gazing off into the quaint abyss, knowing
that dark is right around the corner.
Night arrives, carrying us slowly into
something we have experienced every day
since Morning. But what if each day
we experience is a sped-up version
of a lifetime? What if we are living in
twenty-four hours of
what it means to wake and live and die—
and would we really look at life differently?
Maybe we would move a little slower,
maybe we would rise from bed like it's both
our first and last day on earth.
Maybe we would know the true gift
of living. Maybe we would wake up,
and know we mustn't waste any time.

You will have to ask yourself
many times:

Is this my heart
or my hurt?

I have never met a
cold person
that taught me how to
be warm. I have not
learned much from a
cold person
other than this:
everything stone
eventually cracks.

I saved a cicada from drowning today.
I picked him up, used my breath to blow him dry,
and started to give him a pep-talk.

> *You can do it,*
> *You're going to be okay,*
> *It's just a little water, you're drying off, buddy.*

I gently inched him with my finger,
hoping it would be just the push he needed
to carry on with his day.

I know it's likely he didn't understand.
But it's also likely that he did.
It's very likely that my kindness was just what he
needed.

And even if it wasn't, even if he couldn't understand,
isn't it worth it, just in case?

It's not a coincidence that you were born
exactly the way that you are
with the amount of time that you have.
And if you think that none of this
is connected,
please tell me the exact time
you will be called back to the Earth?
It's funny, we never really have enough time
but have exactly that much,
and still never really know how that can be.

I think I saw
the sadness of the world
before I arrived here.

I have been
swallowing it whole
ever since.

I am constantly propelled by
my capacity to feel both
my sadness and my joy—
as if they were born at the same time.
Together, emerging miraculously,
each entirely different from the other,
but never fully apart.

I'm unsure about most people
until the moment I'm not anymore.
I cried over the way the sun felt and then
we ended up parting ways forever.
In that moment, I knew I would never
feel that same kindness with you and
it was a no brainer:
I must be cautious with my soul.
The sun taught me to go (and stay)
where the warmth is.
I'm just sorry it took me so long
to learn her language.

Maybe we're not meant to find resolve for every internal battle we face. Certainly not all at once and never in any specific time frame. Maybe some battles come with us because we'll need their teachings again someday. Maybe it's more about learning to love ourselves in the midst of hurt and showing up exactly as we are in the moment.

Today, I thought about my sadness.
I remembered all the times I had felt it,
experienced it, drowned in it,
let it swallow me whole.
I realize that is all I do—
think about my sadness,
without ever allowing myself to
work through it.

I can never seem to let things go.
I get stuck on a problem, or a specific
detail of a situation
and run for the hills with it.

When I get to the hills,
hurried and out of breath,
I stare my grievance in the eye.
I wait for its jaw to open in anger
and then walk straight into
the mouth of denial.

Maybe sometimes it's easier to surrender
than it is to put up a fight.

The throat of control leaves no survivors.

Maybe the answer is not what we're looking for.
Maybe we're just desperate to know that
all of this means more than
a fleeting moment in our memory.
Maybe, at our very core,
we just cling to the hope that
we have mattered here;
that something outside of ourselves
cares about our existence just as much as
we care about everything else.
Because it would be silly, right?
To spend most of our time worrying—
if it weren't going to be remembered?

And, in a magical turn of events,
I chose me.

And nothing was the same after that.

Do you know how deeply
you must love something
to have already lived through
its ending in your mind?

Any love I've ever experienced
is a delicate balance between
grief and bliss.

I know that I deserve good things.
But on my worst days, it's hard to convince myself.
I've been a thousand different people
and haven't been so fond of most of them.
I don't know if I ever expected to meet this "me."
Who I am now is not who I was,
but is who I will always strive to be.
I've taken the parts that I love and wrote them in the sky,
french-kissed the open air and ran wild
for the sake of keeping her.
I don't want to destroy her, no,
I want to make her better.
I can't afford to lose any more of me.

Please do not let your empathy become a fixed trait. Give it room to expand, to transform, to take on new heights. Consider it a practice you are always perfecting. You are an ever-growing emotional power. Do not forget that the space around you (and within you) doesn't have to feel like a void. You deserve to protect your empathy as much as you feel it.

Right now you are reading words,
and when I write them,
all it takes is letters to words to lines—
and because you can read them,
you understand.
You understand what you have been taught.
At the beginning of everything,
someone created meaning for what you are seeing.
If we were to strip away all that we know
about words and their meanings,
there would be nothing to interpret.
Nothing to read, just an observation
and a feeling.
And isn't that what poetry is for, anyway?

I don't know how to feel without
letting it grow its own heartbeat
in my stomach.

I don't know how to panic
without it bringing me
to my knees.

I don't know how to love
without properly
feeling all its opposites first.

Compassion goes
both ways. I give you mine
but I always have to ask
for yours. I want to be
human enough for you.
I want the grace of
taking off my mask
and falling short.

I fear, at times, there isn't
anything new to write—
only the sound of a
crumbling world, too many
hearts breaking in unison.
Heartbreak is a part of life?
No.
Not this kind.

A mile from my house sat a hidden
gem that everyone passed by twice a day
but never cared enough to notice.
Between an old factory and an abandoned house
sat a large rock and open sky.
You wouldn't think much of it.
But when my chest would tighten and
my bones would shake, I'd sneak out
as the stars whispered my name and walk
the mile to sit there. I loved that nobody
loved it the way I did. I love that nobody
knew. And that is where my sadness grew.
Upon this rock four times my size,
I learned who I was, and what was important,
and I felt like the open sky understood
that I was in danger but never blamed me.
I think, for once, the darkness wanted to save me.

Thought:

A weight. A mirror. A choice.

When I am alone,
I am me.
I am this skin and these bones
and these thoughts that no one knows.
But as soon as I venture
outside of myself,
I become a spun-out version
of what everyone expects of me.
And that's the last person
I'd ever want to be.

I will never see a time
where I'm not
in my head.

Stop trying to fix me
and just love me
instead.

It wouldn't have been right, you know?
It wouldn't have been right to
hurt you back.
I guess when the people who are supposed
to teach you right from wrong
do you so unthinkably wrong,
you get to decide:
Is this my heart, too?
Or do I steer so clear of your ways,
that I allow other people to hurt me
and be the only one who pays?
I've never had the heart to hurt
someone else's.
In my mind I have thought of all the ways
to tear your life apart—
but my heart wouldn't ever dare.
It only knows how it feels
to keep adding more hurt to an
already-overwhelming pile.
And, well,
I just couldn't do that to you.
I couldn't do that to anyone.
So I'll pay the price. I'll take the hurt
and wish you well.
Maybe someday it will be
an asset. Something I can use.
I learned that from you.

I have spent the majority of my life
making sure that people know that I love them.
I spent a fraction of that time asking
if they loved me just the same.
So who's really to blame?

Ever since I could remember, I've tried
to find the meaning of my existence
in anything outside of myself; I've asked
too many strangers and too many stars.
I remember asking at seven.
I asked at twelve again.
I kept asking as the years went on.

At first, I thought:
I exist to save everybody else.
That is my purpose.
I am an Indigo Child, an experiment
from another planet sent here
to bear the worst of the world
and absorb the pain so others
would be spared it.

So when the world smacks me,
I take it.
Better me than them,
I'm not supposed to be here, anyway,
so it's almost like it doesn't count.

Sometimes, I can't see the
person inside of me that
people claim to love because
the world taught her that
she had to stay hidden
in order to survive.

It's hard to know who I am
when who I am
always swallows me whole.

The thing about being the person who
perpetually carries everything in their heart
is that you will never leave it,
even if I want you to.
Even if I must leave, I take you with me,
tuck your fears behind my ear and
put a pin in it when they're in the way.
Even when you hurt me,
I am still hoping you are not
hurting for the years to come—
hoping that somewhere down the line,
on a random Tuesday,
you understand that the way you mattered to me
changed me irrevocably,
I carried you with me all this time.
And that's the thing about being the person
who perpetually carries everything in their heart:
You will always be loved and I
will always just be the carrier:
a collector of overlooked memories,
always hoping to be seen.

The version of yourself
that you are so eager to meet
hides underneath you all along.
It is there—it is actually
guiding you. Its only
requirement is that you
listen.

I have died on countless occasions—
at the shaky hand of cruelty and ignorance.
I sometimes wonder if I exist solely
to teach others what it is like to
lose unwavering love. I wonder if
all I'm good for is a lesson
no one thinks about twice.

Maybe this isn't what you wanted but
it's what you got. I'd like to tell you that
it's unfortunate (because it is), but
I hope it showed you the truth. I hope
it unveiled so many secrets—
some you will have to learn to undeny,
others you will have to say aloud.
The world can't hide from you now,
because you know its secrets.
This isn't the time to be vindictive.
The truth is that no human being
should ever be a secret
you bury that deep.

You cannot hold another person's
jacket for too long before finally
putting it on yourself.

This is what I mean when I tell you:
Be careful what you carry.

You have not lived until music
has slowed the fast track of your heart.
Until the inevitable change of the
day's sky has altered your circadian rhythm
and you're up all night creating
mausoleums out of lead. You have not lived
until you've met someone whose vibrance
inspires a decade of gratitude. Until you've
slowed down just enough to think about all
the small things that were once alive, out there,
somewhere, dead and nobody knows. Until
you've found them, and held a moment of
silence. Silence. You have not lived until
you have lived in the silence and found
peace there. Until everything you've ever
known about yourself becomes concrete
and vulnerable and harmonious.

You will be easily swayed by your emotions. But please know that your truth can be found in all that remains hidden. Look inward and ask what you are keeping tucked away. Ask what is locked. Open it and allow it to have a voice. You are protecting others from the pain you once felt, but you are also taking it on for yourself. You don't need any more of that pain. You have enough. So, sing, speak, cry—however it wants to come out. But please remember: anyone worth protecting this way would never ask you to bury what burdens you.

If you consider how little time we have
and then consider the
abundance of time we still have—
they end up canceling each other out.
And then all we're really left with
is the Time right Here and Now.

We come into this world
learning how to love each other.
Let us not leave this world
wishing that we *had*.

I am not calculated, I am traumatized.
It's an easy mistake to make.
The truth is that you haven't walked
my same walk. You only know the length.
I could tell you stories,
ones you assuredly won't believe—
ask you to walk along with me.
But unless you have heard every instance or
felt every neglect, you'll never be in my head.
I am a human that has lived
several lives in three decades—
some mine,
and some not.
It must be so easy to misunderstand me
if you have only lived this one.
I could name a thousand people
who never truly saw me for who I was.
And if I'm being honest,
I never really let them.

Collective wounds
require
collective balms.

Sometimes, my self-care is
self-preservation. And sometimes,
that looks a lot like struggle.
This is because I am still learning
how to listen to my body's plea

for calm

and determining what it needs.
Sometimes, I don't get an answer.
But I go to all ends of the Earth
to find what may bring stillness.
I call this devotion. I call this love.
I call this learning,
and it's all for me.

The anglerfish decided that
for her last trick,
she'd ascend to a light she's never seen before.
A light she wasn't sure even existed.
With her final breaths,
her little body swam until
floating atop was an option.
Just to say goodbye—
proving to the world that beautiful
things do come from places
we cannot see.
Proving to the world that you can be
small and undiscovered and still find
a light you didn't know existed.
It may take all of your strength,
but imagine how bright it will be before you go.

Do I let this go,
or do I hold on for dear life?
If we're being honest,
you know it will become
an integral part of me
anyway.

Sometimes
stepping back is helpful
in making a
great leap forward.

I was born to love. My capacity to love was only exacerbated by the immense neglect and pain I had experienced. But that wasn't going to stop me regardless. Even as a child, I knew love was the only answer. I stand in the face of pain, sob through my stomach, and carry it with me so I never forget what it feels like.

I want to love everything, oh, even if it hurts.

The birds talk to each other and
to our ears, it sounds like singing.

Don't tell me that isn't
some sort of inexplicable magic.

Pay attention:

Shine. Lean. Whisper. Scream. Sprout. Fall. Come
alive again when you're ready. Pace. Revival.
It's okay, I forgive you. Nourish me. Take care.
Intentional. Change happens without question.
Stand tall. Roots replanted even when they are
tightly bound. Soothe. Rehabilitate. Impermanence.
Repurpose. Breathe, no worries. See you in the
morning.

Maybe you don't have to stop
worrying, per se. Maybe you
just need to look at the quality
of your worry. Instead of fearing
the inevitable outcomes, maybe we
worry about how we can love
ourselves a little better that day.
Maybe we take the concept and
point it towards ourselves this time—
Make "us" the thing we worry over.
Turn the worry inward until
it becomes care. It is needed there.

It is okay to be a person
who is still healing.
Because the truth is that
we always will be.
It is an "always" practice.
That forever kind of love—
with yourself.

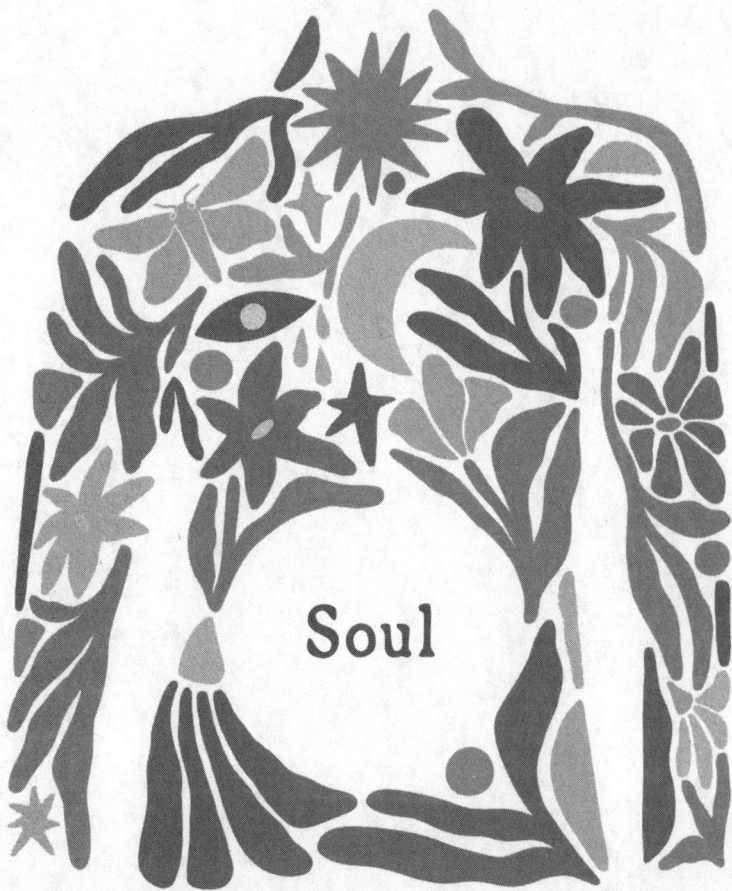

Soul

Why, in even my calmest states,
does it always feel as though my soul
is in perpetual oneness
with devastation?

If you convert your anger to sadness,
that anger will still sit in your body.
And the longer it sits in your body,
the more it plagues your soul.
In body,
In mind,
In soul.

You are way too sensitive.

You have such a deep capacity for emotion.

You're taking this too personally.

I know this feels heavy for you.

We don't have time for this.

Let your emotions stay for as long as they need to.

This isn't about you.

It's okay to feel sad for another person.

I'm not going to sit here while you're emotional.

I'll sit with you in your sadness for as long as you need.

You make me uncomfortable.

I'm not comfortable with my own emotions.

You are weak.

Your capacity to feel is what makes you strong.

No one wants to be around you.

The right people will appreciate this about you.

You're going to make yourself sick.

Make sure you're taking care of yourself, too.

I didn't believe that there was room
on this Earth
for my entire range of emotions
until I started *making* space for them.
Once they started taking up space,
I realized I needed a bigger room.
Eventually, they'll occupy a home.
And the windows will flap their arms
and the roof will echo laughter
throughout the entire neighborhood.
At times, the shutters will bat their
eyes and cry, and the chimney will
blow its smoke. And it will be
the safest place I will ever know.

I was convinced that there was something
irreparably wrong with me,
that my soul was born naturally defective,
and that everyone around me could see it.
I used that as a crutch whenever
life got the better of me, and licked the seal
of my unworthiness with the proof.
But alas, our souls are not the envelopes,
they are the message carefully slipped inside of them.
Some might see the name and rip it up.
But someone is waiting to read it,
to cherish it,
to send their love back.
And the truth is that the Post Office
is a dying love these days,
and it's illegal to open someone else's mail.
If only the same sentiment applied
to the ripping of souls, the crushing of spirit.
Maybe it all has to be dying
for us to really love it.

I always leave a bowl of fruit out in the kitchen.
And sure, it always goes bad but there's
nothing quite like creating an environment
that says:
you're safe here, take me,
you are worthy of this food,
take a tangerine
and stay a while,
we like having you here.
You are worthy in this house.

Someone once told me that
the eyes of a teddy bear are intentionally
made to have a neutral expression,
so that children could project
their own emotions into them
to create a sense of safety and comfort.
"How considerate," I thought,
"That someone knew we would need it."

I didn't know what I was capable of.
I fear that I never really knew
who I was, that I was never given
a fraction of a chance to be great
in this world.
What are the odds? That I'd land
in exactly this life, with not one single
person to really love me,
and end up finding something that
resembles peace?
I'll tell you what: I didn't like the odds.
At some point, I had to scoop myself up
from the basement of rock bottom and
make a way of existing that didn't feel like
dying.

I just know that everything hurt,
and that's who I was. Hurt.
And I didn't want to be Hurt anymore.

The sun is going down and
it happens every night
but today is different.
Today was hard, and the sun still went down—
I felt it touch my skin and came alive again,
if only for a brief moment.
But tomorrow the sun will rise,
and I will feel it on my skin again.
And all of these days combined
are a perfectly beautiful collection
of proof that I

have survived.

I will never beg you to care,
because that isn't real.
I have begged far too many times—
enough to know that anything
worth my soul won't feel like
desperation.

Everyone I know is hurting. And rightfully so—
This world took hope and slashed it at the ankles.
How do we know which way is up? Which way is down?
Am I wrong or right? Is this good or bad?
I have 87 alarms in my phone and not a single one
does the trick. I have wounds to lick.
I think the world is bleeding and my lips aren't full
and my body is not the same as it was
and an online doctor told me the broccoli I eat
doesn't have nutrients because you must let it sit after
you cut it.
But I'm hungry, and I'm tired,
and most of the country would rather me die
than be in love with an angel for 99 years.
And it's time to eat again,
the laundry has been at the door (crying and toppled
over each other)—
I say it's for *comfort*.
        (. . . And how do I find that?)
I stayed inside for four years and all I got was more
of the same
mental disorder. But nobody wants to hear about that.
My head is contaminated, and my body is craving
something I don't think it will ever find in this lifetime.
And the deep loneliness won't be cured
by a 50-minute broccoli dish or figuring out
if my cortisol is too high.
When did people stop meaning something to each other?
And where the hell are their heads?
You can be everything right and still hurt like hell.
The questions we are asking are too expensive.
And the price? Is you.

If I could go back in time
and tell little me one thing
that would change the course
of my entire life,

it would be this:
Cry your heart out.
Because all that harboring
is going to eat you from the inside out
before the worms ever do.

I love people with a knife
already buried in my back.
So that before they ever have
the chance to hurt me,
I have already
good and well
done it to myself.
Call me pessimistic but,
this is how we survive out here.
It is survival of the sensitives.

Pretend that everything you've ever felt was placed into a bag.
Your every worry, thought, emotion (your own and the ones you absorb). Your empathy, your perspective, the tears you have cried. The heartbreak you've carried from people you've long moved on from. The tears, the panic, the boundless amount of beauty you have seen. The potential you see from people and the world. You'd need a pretty big vessel to put all of this into, right?

That's how large your soul is.

I engulfed myself in other people's darkest shadows.
I would dive right in with every intention
to pull out even the smallest beam of light I could find.
But it occurred to me that the longer I searched,
the deeper I had gotten.
And somewhere along the way, my light went out.

You were given
this exact soul of yours
to be constantly curious
about its complexity.
You do not need to search
for all the ways that it
needs to be fixed. What if it was
meant to be so full that
it became tangible? What if
your soul is the living embodiment
of what it means to experience life?
A soul that deep is meant
to be felt.

I don't need to be well-received.
The world performs too much of that.
Instead, I'd hope you'd ask me to be soft,
to allow my deepest pain and
deepest love
to rise to the surface,
and weave them together like palm fronds.
Let them be my roof, my blanket,
my living proof that being human
doesn't need to be the life-long
death sentence we've made it out to be.
Let me laugh and cry and ask you
to hold my hand.
Let's sit together under the sky and
forget everything on land.

I was tough—
And I wasn't designed for it.
That is the disconnect.

The sensitive suffer.
They suffer and they
survive,
and extend love farther
than your eyes could dream,
even as they actively hurt.
And then they suffer, yet again,
for all of it.

I'm going to tell you something that was once told to me, something I've never forgotten. You are a sensitive soul who loves harder than most people can comprehend. And because of this, you need to find someone who loves you *more* than you love them. Because if we're being honest, it's not entirely possible—not in our brain, at least. So when you're out there, loving people with every ounce of yourself that has ever existed, remember not to settle until you find someone who loves you even harder. Because that is the only way we will ever feel truly seen: when all our sensitive is loved and returned back to us in a way only we could deeply understand.

How do I heal if I have never fully
recovered from most things? I have
never quite found the way to cut
the cord of the strumming inside of me,
dull and raw and so out-of-tune.

I have yet to find a way
through anything
that doesn't put a
hole in me.

Friedrich Nietzsche once wrote
that if you gaze long enough
into the abyss, the abyss will
gaze back into you.

He never mentioned what it means
to stare into the abyss and already
recognize its face.

I cry—
And each tear is a
desperate "I'm sorry"
to my Self.
And a new world
opens up in my chest.
One where I can be
in my body.
One where I accept
the apologies.

My mother always taught me that
once you give something away,
It's rude to take it back—
That it's a known rule:
Once it's gone, it's no longer yours.
I think I carried this too deeply.
I think I gave myself to people
and never thought to consider asking for "me" back.

Your wounds are not your end-all.
Do you hear me?
Your wounds are not your end-all.

You are never behind in life.
But I can tell you what you are behind.
You are behind the love,
behind the hope,
the empathy and compassion;
behind the glimmer of joy
still left in this world.
You are the one behind it.
Because without you,
this world would be much more
behind
than it already is, for a lot of people.
We're holding onto every single
sliver of a moment that brings
peace—
so, in a world that needs a rebirth,
you are perfectly ahead of schedule.

You can't force your heart
to mend until
you feel everything that
it asks you to feel.
Then it will cooperate.
But first you must be willing
to lie in the mess.

The right people
will never question
that heart of yours.

Do not apologize for taking extra time
to breathe the air. For retreating when
you feel like a shell of yourself, for
loving people who cannot see you.
Do not apologize for being gentle
in a world that does nothing but
ask you to be anything else.
The depth you are able to feel
is not a lack, love,
but a muscle.

A childhood friend of mine once snuck me into a secret part of her property where she discovered a honeysuckle tree. It was nestled between her mom's garden and a grass alleyway, climbing up the edge of a fence. It smelled like nothing I had ever experienced before, and I was positive that this flower was not from this world. She taught me to pick off a flower, pull out the middle, and suck the honey out from what was left over. This memory lives in my head like a warm summer where nothing else matters. I knew I would carry those moments and that lesson with me everywhere I went. But somewhere along the way, I forgot the point of it all. I would stare in awe at the honeysuckle bush in my mind but never touch it. My entire life has been a reclaiming of what it means to stumble upon something beautiful and reteaching my heart that I'm allowed to partake in the sweetness.

My spirit won't allow me
to carry hate in my heart.
So I will take yours,
And hang it with my flowers
to dry out.

Maybe the void is just a longing;
for what was, or is,
or should have always been.
A void that sits cross-legged
between your ribs and your stomach,
swirling around in the hopes that
life will hear its moaning and deliver.
A space that waits for the day
it will take its first and final breath.
One you have tirelessly tried to fill
with no relief,

yet.

I know that you give slivers of your soul to each person that asks for your attention. I also know that to ask you to change that would be asking you to change who you are at your core. And we don't want to do that. But I will ask you why you love to give, but never to yourself. You are excluding yourself from the mix. You know that there is an endless amount of love in that body of yours and you do not save any for your own heart. Half of the beauty of giving is to be able to see yourself as somebody worth receiving. Did you forget that you are human, too?

When you feel yourself
withering away: pause.
Take whatever is left and
go elsewhere. Go inward.
Go find your medicine.
Nothing is worth
the wilting.

I'm not supportive,
not fond of nor proud
of my self-abuse.
I carry untold debt to my soul.
It is the least I can do—
to be gentle with it.

If I bring anything to this world,
I need it to be this:

I hope that you feel loved around me.

The world will always demand
more of you. It will grind you
to a pulp and drink you for breakfast
if you don't first find a way to
keep yourself whole.

In case your brain is telling you otherwise:

You matter. People are not better off without you, even though they've treated you in a way that exacerbates that feeling. I know you have been hurt so often that you've lost count, and I know that hurt piles up. It's easy to find meaning in the hurt and assume the blame. The truth is that you're not responsible for how another person moves through the world or how they treat other people. It's almost never personal, we just take it as so. Because sometimes, we just need an answer and when we don't have one, we become the answer. But most of the time, it has nothing to do with you or the love you give. A misalignment between people does not equate to your worth or what you bring to this world. In fact, it is required even more.

You took me away from myself.
And I spent all my time asking
if I could somehow give you more.
You kept
taking and I kept
allowing
and somewhere along this very devastating line,
I realized it wasn't me that you wanted.
It was my heart. You wanted it
as your own, something to mimic.
And because I could never instill that
in you, you became angry and
I became empty.
I fell apart right where you left me.
And from the moment I got up,
you have always resented me.

On days where you forget
that the world holds more than pain,
search for the quiet. The quiet
holds glimmers that the noise
could never reveal. Search for it
everywhere. Let it take you in.
The quiet is a soft friend.
And where there is love and kindness
and softness and vulnerability,
there is strength and wisdom
and
I can feel myself mending.

I release my soul from hanging onto
anything that asks me to abandon it.
I choose to embrace my heart
even when it feels defeated.
Where there is the truth of you—
all else runs its natural course.

Your inner peace should never
be up for debate or negotiation.
There is not a settlement
to be made, no loophole
for others to find.

Your inner peace stands at the front,
an investment in self—
but never a transaction.

Oh,
to be understood at the very core of things.
To be loved.
To be changed.
To be seen.
To be safe.

Acknowledgments

Writing books has been a dream of mine that I never imagined could be achieved. When I wrote my first book, it sat in my phone for over ten years because I never thought it could amount to much. I didn't believe in the possibility of dreams, but taking a chance on myself changed the trajectory of my life.

I want to thank my agent, Steven Harris, for believing in me and my work from the moment we met. You advocate for me, you lift me up, and you have become family to me. I am grateful to my entire team at HarperOne for bringing such a sensitive book to life and believing in the importance of my poetry. My editor, Ryan Amato, for working so hard with me to create the most amazing collection and for always advocating for queer voices in the publishing world. Yung Pueblo, an inspiration and a dear friend, thank you for seeing me and my capability before I fully saw myself—your support of me over the years has encouraged me to keep putting meaningful work into the world. Much gratitude to my wonderful friend and cover designer, Natalia Skeba: you have worked with me since the beginning, and we connected instantly. You have been a light in my life ever since! Thank you for designing the cover of *Bellyache* and bringing this collection to life with your talent.

I also want to thank the friends I have made within the online poetry space, who are far too many to name, but without whom I would not have had the courage to keep trying. Last but certainly not least, I want to thank my spouse. Not only have you healed and loved so many parts of me, but you have encouraged me to become the version of myself that I feel most proud of. Without you, these books would still be sitting in my phone, waiting to see the light of day, and I would still be hiding from the world. Thank you for loving me in a way that makes me love myself enough to be seen by the world.

About the Author

Brianna Pastor (she/they) is a queer writer, empath, advocate, and author of the poetry collections *Good Grief* and *Bellyache*. Dedicated to helping others recognize their worth regardless of circumstances, Pastor centers her poetry around mental health, childhood trauma, and what it means to heal—with sensitivity and love at the root of all things. Brianna resides in New Jersey with her spouse and their cat, Boogie.

To read more, connect with Brianna:

Instagram: @briannapastor
Threads: @briannapastor
TikTok: @briannapastorpoetry